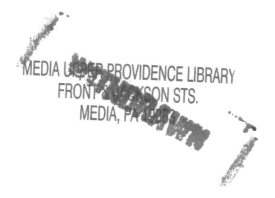

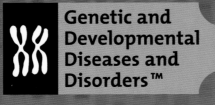

Genetic and Developmental Diseases and Disorders™

Sickle Cell Anemia

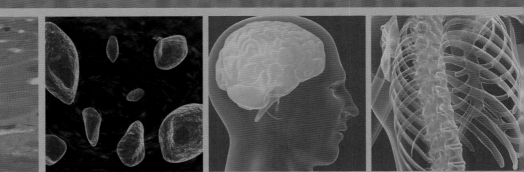

Judy Monroe Peterson

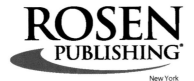

ROSEN PUBLISHING®

New York

To my husband, Dave, for all his wonderful help and support

Published in 2009 by The Rosen Publishing Group, Inc.
29 East 21st Street, New York, NY 10010
www.rosenpublishing.com

First Edition

Library of Congress Cataloging-in-Publication Data

Peterson, Judy Monroe.
Sickle cell anemia / Judy Monroe Peterson.—1st ed.
        p.cm.—(Genetic and developmental diseases and disorders)
Includes bibliographical references and index.
ISBN-13: 978-1-4042-1851-2 (library binding)
1. Sickle cell anemia. I. Title.
RC641.7.S5P48 2009
616.1'527—dc22

                                                              2007040003

Manufactured in Malaysia

On the cover: Background: An electron micrograph shows human red blood cells on the wall of a blood vessel. Foreground: Sickle cells, the red blood cells that are shaped like crescents, can block small blood vessels, which results in less blood reaching that part of the body.

Contents

Introduction 4

1 Sickle Cell Anemia in History 7

2 Understanding Sickle Cells 15

3 Living with Sickle Cell Anemia 25

4 Researching New Treatments 35

5 Hope for the Future 41

Timeline 49

Glossary 52

For More Information 54

For Further Reading 57

Bibliography 58

Index 62

Introduction

One drop of your blood contains millions of red blood cells. Red blood cells travel throughout your body to deliver oxygen and take away waste from your tissues. These cells get their color from hemoglobin, which is the chemical in red blood cells that allows them to carry oxygen around the body.

Red blood cells look like doughnuts. They are flat, soft, and round and have a dimple in the middle. They move quickly through tiny blood tubes called capillaries in all parts of the body. The bodies of people with sickle cell anemia sometimes form red blood cells that look like bananas, or sickles. These long red blood cells are hard and sticky and have pointed ends. Instead of flowing freely through the capillaries, the sickle cells have the tendency to bunch up. Some break apart. Bunching up or breaking apart slows or stops the flow of blood. Then cells do not get enough oxygen, and waste products from the cells cannot be taken away. The lack of oxygen and buildup of

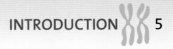

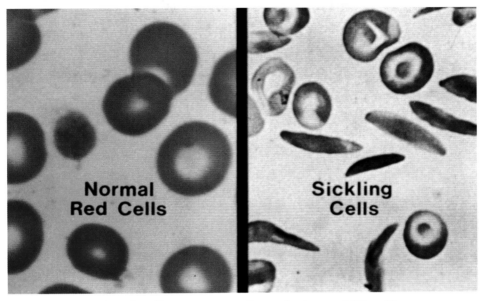

Normal red blood cells are smooth and shaped like discs or doughnuts, but without a hole in the middle. Sickle cells bend into the shape of sickles or crescent moons.

waste products in the tissues cause great pain and can even cause death.

Sickle cell anemia is a genetic disease of the blood. It is caused by a biological defect in one gene of a person. Genes are the elements in cells that carry the information that determines traits, such as hair or eye color. In sickle cell anemia, a defect in the gene controls how hemoglobin is made. This defect can be passed from parents to their children.

What is it like to have sickle cell anemia? Maya Priest recalled that she did many of the same activities as other kids when she was in grade school. However, she always had to drink a lot of water, and she could not play in the snow. She hurt all over when it was cold. Starting in the seventh grade, she missed a lot of school because she hurt constantly. A tutor came to her house to help her with schoolwork. When she felt better, Priest would go out with friends. Sometimes, she could not keep up with her friends because she felt tired and needed to rest. Today, she has a job. She still has to drink a lot of water and take her medicine every day.

Priest has constant pain. The pain is worse some days and not so bad on other days. When the pain is mild, she stays at home to rest. When the pain gets severe, she goes to the hospital for treatment. Sometimes, she stays in the hospital for a week or more. Her pain affects her studies and work.

Maya Priest is not alone. According to the National Institutes of Health (NIH), about 72,000 Americans are living with the disease of sickle cell anemia. Most are African Americans. Some Hispanic Americans also have the disease. The NIH estimates that millions of people worldwide have sickle cell anemia. It is most common in people who live by large bodies of water in warm areas of the world.

1

No one knows exactly when sickle cell anemia was first reported. Sickle cell anemia is a blood disease. Ancient people did not understand the parts of blood, what blood does, or how the body makes blood. They did not have the tools, such as microscopes, to look at blood and to understand it.

Ancient people did not know the cause of sickle cell anemia. However, they saw children suffering from the painful disease. Sickle cell anemia is more common in Africa than on any other continent. African tribes called the disease by various names. The Twi tribe named it *ahututuo*. The Ga tribe called it *chwecheechwe*. Another name was *nuidudui* from the Ewe tribe, and the Fante tribe called it *nwiiwii*.

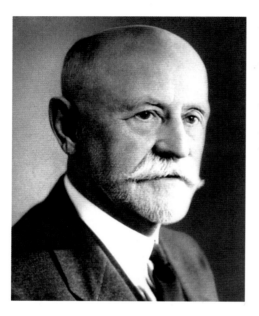

James B. Herrick, an American doctor, wrote an article about a person who had odd red blood cells. In his report, Herrick included photos of the cells and was the first to call the unusual cells "sickle-shaped."

Some African tribes named the disease from the cries of pain that children made. Other tribes used terms such as "body chewing" or "body biting" to tell about the pain that people have with sickle cell anemia. In Cameroon, people called the disease *adep*, meaning "beaten up." This name tells how people with sickle cell anemia feel.

Many babies with sickle cell anemia died without a doctor's care. A West African tribe called the children who died soon after birth *ogbanjes*. This term means "children who come and go." They believed a demon, or evil spirit, was trying to be born into a family with *ogbanje* babies. They thought the babies died to save the family from the demon.

Until the 1900s, most children who had sickle cell anemia did not live to become adults. Doctors seldom saw children with the disease. When they did, they did not know that this disease was different from other common diseases. The symptoms of sickle cell anemia are often similar to those of other tropical diseases. Early doctors did not know to look at the blood of people with sickle cell anemia.

Early Discoveries

An American doctor, R. Lebby, wrote the first modern description of sickle cell anemia in 1846 in an article titled "Case of Absence of the Spleen." The spleen is a large organ in the body to the left of the stomach. It stores blood and destroys old red blood cells. Lebby had looked at the organs in an African American slave who had died. The dead man did not have a spleen. The doctor wrote about this observation and other medical conditions concerning the dead man's body.

The next published reports of sickle cell disease were in African medical articles. These articles started to appear in the 1870s. Scientists then began to look for causes of the disease.

Progress in the study of sickle cell anemia came in 1910. That year, Dr. James B. Herrick published an article about the disease. Herrick was a heart doctor living in Chicago, Illinois. Walter Clement Noel, a twenty-year-old student from the West Indies, came to Herrick for treatment. Noel had difficulty breathing, stomach pains, and pain in his muscles. He had open sores, or ulcers, on his legs. He always felt tired and had anemia, meaning a low red blood cell count. Anemia, which causes a person to feel tired, can happen because of a variety of disorders or diseases.

Herrick wrote down all the symptoms. He then looked under a microscope at Noel's blood. He observed some unusual circumstances. For instance, he did not see many normal, round red blood cells. Instead, he saw long, thin red blood cells. He thought the cells looked like sickles. Herrick

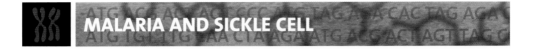

MALARIA AND SICKLE CELL

The areas of the world that have high numbers of people with the sickle cell trait also have high rates of malaria. Malaria is a tropical disease caused by a parasite carried by mosquitoes. A theory from the 1940s is that the genetic mutation of sickle cell trait occurred thousands of years ago and increased the chance that sickle cell carriers could survive malaria. Survivors then passed the mutation to their offspring. The trait became established in areas where malaria was common.

wondered if the strange red blood cells were the cause of the young man's anemia. He published photos of the strange cells so that others could see them. Herrick was the first person to call the cells "sickle-shaped" and is credited as the first person to describe sickle cell anemia.

Over the next fifteen years, doctors published articles about other people with the strange cells and similar symptoms. In 1917, Victor Emmel, another American doctor, treated an African American woman for anemia. Emmel looked at the woman's blood under a microscope and saw many sickle cells. He then looked at blood from her father. He found some sickle cells, but not as many as he saw in the daughter's blood. Interestingly, the father was healthy and showed no symptoms of anemia. Emmel also discovered that several siblings of the woman had died from anemia.

Genetic Link?

Based on these articles and other published research, scientists began to think that sickle cell anemia was an inherited disease because it seemed to run in families. Many of these families were of African descent. They also found that sickling, or having sickle cells in the blood, was more common in African countries around the equator and in parts of India. However, scientists could not say why the disease was found in mostly tropical areas.

In 1923, John Huck at Johns Hopkins University Medical School in Baltimore, Maryland, looked into the idea that the disease is inherited. He traced sickle cell anemia in two different families through multiple generations. His discovery suggested that there was a genetic link.

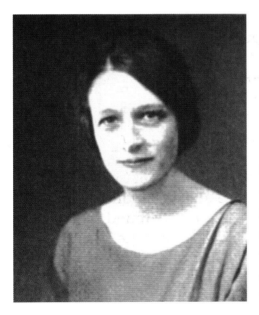

Elizabeth Gillespie *left* and E. Vernon Hahn worked together at Indiana University School of Medicine to discover the relationship of sickle-shaped cells and low levels of oxygen in the blood.

The Strange Red Blood Cells

Beginning in the 1920s, scientists tried to discover why red blood cells in some people were shaped like sickles. Two scientists at Indiana University School of Medicine in Indianapolis studied the effects of oxygen on the blood. E. Vernon Hahn and Elizabeth Gillespie showed that red blood cells became sickle-shaped if oxygen in the blood was very low. Hahn first used the term "sickle cell trait" to describe healthy people who had some sickle cells. Hahn and Gillespie published an article about their work in 1927.

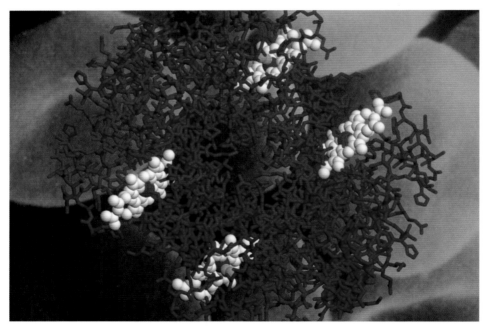

Hemoglobin appears as red in this computer model. Hemoglobin, a protein, is the substance in red blood cells that carries oxygen from the lungs to tissues in the body.

During the 1940s, scientists made important discoveries about the cause of sickling. Irving Sherman, then a student at Johns Hopkins, found that the sickling of red blood cells is caused by a change in hemoglobin. Hemoglobin is the part of red blood cells that carries oxygen.

From 1945 to 1948, Dr. Janet Watson of the Long Island College of Medicine in Brooklyn, New York, studied sickle cells. She looked at the blood of more than 200 African American mothers and their newborn babies. She found that the newborns had few sickle cells. The mothers had many more sickle cells. Watson wondered if the difference in the number of sickle cells was due to different types of hemoglobin, which are different in adults and newborns. She tested some newborns until they were four-month-old babies. At that age, the babies had much more sickling. Watson thought that sickling of cells begins when a newborn's hemoglobin is replaced by different hemoglobin. She published her work in 1948.

That same year, another scientist, Dr. Linus Pauling, published his findings about a medical breakthrough that he had made during work on sickle cell anemia and hemoglobin. His research supported the work of Watson. Scientists were now unlocking the secrets of sickle cell anemia.

Myths and Facts

Myth: Sickle cell anemia can be transmitted to, or caught by, other people.
Fact: Sickle cell anemia is not contagious. It is an inherited disease and is passed from parent to child.

Myth: Only African Americans have sickle cell anemia.
Fact: Sickle cell can affect people of many different back grounds, including African Americans and people of Hispanic, Mediterranean, Middle Eastern, and South Asian descent. According to the National Institutes of Health, the disease affects mainly African Americans. It occurs in about 1 in every 500 African American births, and in about 1 out of every 1,000 to 1,400 Hispanic American births.

Myth: If you have sickle cell anemia, you cannot prevent a pain crisis.
Fact: You can help prevent a pain crisis by following a healthy lifestyle. Get regular exercise and plenty of rest, eat healthy meals, and drink lots of water. Because lung infections are common in people with the disease, do not smoke or be in a smoky room. Contact your doctor at the first signs of an infection, such as a fever or difficulty breathing. Wear warm clothes in cold weather and inside air-conditioned rooms. Do not swim in cold water or be at high altitudes. Only travel in an airplane if the cabin is pressurized.

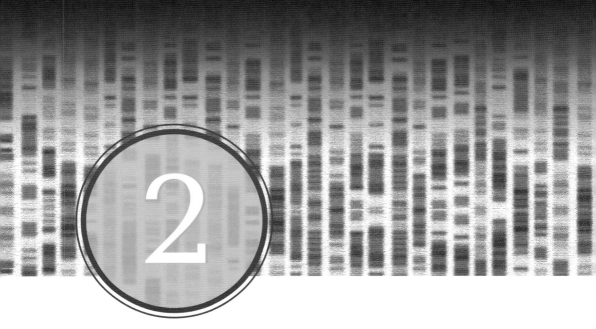

Understanding Sickle Cells

Modern research into sickle cell anemia began in 1945 when Linus Pauling, an American chemist, became curious about sickle cells. He wondered if sickle cell anemia was a disease of the hemoglobin molecules. A red blood cell is made up mostly of these molecules. In 1948, Pauling published his groundbreaking research. He found that sickling occurs when red blood cells have abnormal hemoglobin. Pauling called the hemoglobin "S" for sickle.

He also discovered that hemoglobin S is much less soluble, or able to be dissolved, than normal hemoglobin. When Pauling packed hemoglobin S inside red blood cells, it formed tiny crystals. The crystals pushed through the membranes of the cells, causing the cells to become shaped like sickles. Pauling was the

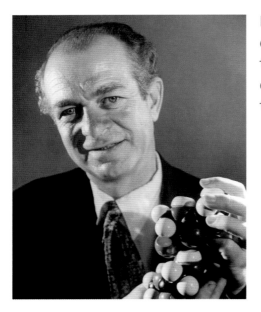

Linus Pauling, an American chemist, was the first to discover that sickle cell anemia was caused by a small change in the structure of hemoglobin.

first to show that the cause of a disease was due to a change in protein structure. Meanwhile, other scientists were researching how the disease was transmitted from parents to their offspring.

Inheritance of Sickle Cell Anemia

The science of genetics began in the mid-1800s. However, the mechanisms of how traits were passed from parents to their offspring were not well understood until a century later. In the first half of the 1900s, scientists established that deoxyribonucleic acid (DNA) carried genetic information. Genetic information is transmitted from parents to their offspring by chromosomes, which are in the nuclei, or central cores, of cells. Chromosomes are structures made of DNA and proteins. DNA is genetic material that contains instructions for life.

Scientists found that DNA contained four nucleotide bases: adenine (A), thymine (T), cytosine (C), and guanine (G). Genes

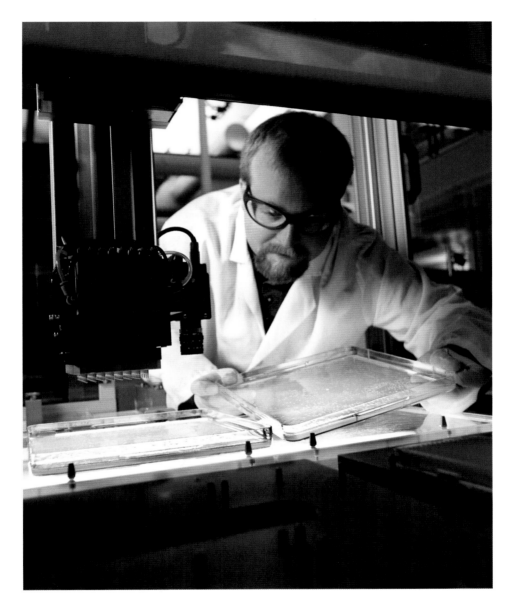

This scientist, who is a researcher for the Human Genome Project, is using a sequencing machine to work on finding the sequence of the genes in human DNA. DNA is the molecule that controls the growth and development of all organisms.

are made of different combinations of the four bases. In England in 1953, scientists James Watson and Francis Crick, along with Rosalind Franklin and Maurice Wilkins, discovered the three-dimensional structure of DNA. DNA is made up of two strands of bases that wind around each other in a double helix, like a spiral staircase.

During this time, Vernon Ingram and J. A. Hunt, two scientists in Cambridge, England, were researching the hemoglobin protein. In 1956, they mapped out the amino acid sequence of sickle cell hemoglobin. An amino acid is a molecule that makes up protein. The important findings of Ingram and Hunt demonstrated that the amino acids of normal hemoglobin and hemoglobin S differ by only one amino acid. This meant that a single mutation in one gene produces hemoglobin S.

Sequencing the Human Genome

Genes are segments of DNA and are located at specific places on a chromosome. Every gene carries instructions on how to make a specific protein. Proteins are the main substances that make up our bodies. A gene or a combination of genes has the instructions for a trait, such as hair color, eye color, height, or face shape. Heredity is the study of how traits are passed from parents to their offspring.

Most cells in the body contain two copies of each chromo-some. One copy comes from the mother, and one comes from the father. Sperm and egg cells contain only one copy of each chromosome. Sperm and egg cells are formed during meiosis. In the process of meiosis, the pairs of chromosomes are copied and then line up at opposite ends of the cell's nucleus. The cell divides twice, forming four cells. Sperm and egg cells are formed, each containing half of each chromosome pair.

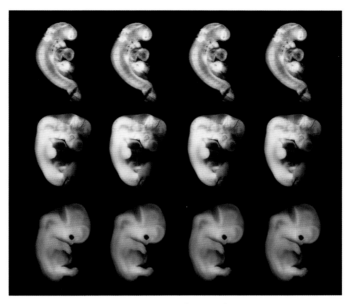

The development of a human embryo from twenty-nine days old to fifty-six days old is shown in this photo. After eight weeks, an embryo is called a fetus.

When a sperm and an egg cell join, an embryo is formed. The embryo receives one half of each pair of its chromosomes from its mother and one half from its father.

To identify the cause of genetic diseases such as sickle cell anemia, scientists needed to establish the location of each gene, the exact arrangement of its nucleotide bases, and the protein it codes for. The invention of techniques to sequence genes made this work possible. To sequence genes, scientists use chemicals to separate the gene into its bases. Then they identify their order. American scientists Allan Maxam and Walter Gilbert and British scientist Fred Sanger independently developed the first process for gene sequencing in 1977.

In the mid-1990s, sequencing of DNA became much faster with new, automated methods. In 1990 in the United States, the

Human Genome Project began to map the location of all the genes on human chromosomes. The project was to finish by 2005. However, another project met this goal by June 2000. This project was started by the American doctor J. Craig Venter, the Applera Corporation, and the company they founded, Celera Genomics.

GENETIC CHANGES OF HEMOGLOBIN IN SICKLE CELL ANEMIA

An embryo, a fetus, and an adult make three different types of hemoglobin. The three types of hemoglobin have the same three parts: heme, alpha globin chains, and beta globin chains. Sickle hemoglobin occurs from a genetic change in the beta globin part of adult hemoglobin. The beta globin gene is located on chromosome 11. The change occurs on codon (position) 6 of the beta globin gene. The amino acid valine is substituted for the amino acid glutamic acid.

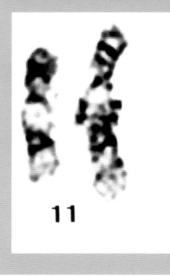

11

People have forty-six chromosomes in each cell. The chromosomes are divided into twenty-three pairs. Two copies of chromosome 11, one copy inherited from each parent, form one of the pairs.

Who Gets Sickle Cell Anemia?

Sometimes, one gene in a chromosome has a mutation in its sequence, and a new trait develops. A different form of the gene for the hemoglobin protein in red blood cells causes sickle cell anemia. One amino acid in the protein is replaced by a different amino acid. The gene that affects the hemoglobin protein also affects the shape of the cells, causing red blood cells to become sickle-shaped.

This type of gene mutation is typically inherited from a mother and father who have the sickle cell trait or anemia. In 1978, British scientist Richard Anthony Flavell mapped the human genes that code for hemoglobin. His work showed that sickle cell anemia is a single gene disorder that is caused by a mutation in the DNA sequence of one gene.

Most people have two normal copies of the beta globin gene. This gene makes the normal beta globin in adult hemoglobin. People with sickle cell trait have one normal beta globin gene and one sickle cell beta globin gene. They make normal and sickle hemoglobin in about the same amounts. Although people with sickle cell trait (called carriers) can pass along the mutated gene to their children, they themselves usually are healthy.

When both a mother and a father are carriers of sickle cell trait, their baby has three possible inheritances: in each pregnancy, the baby has a 25 percent chance of inheriting two sickle cell genes and will then have sickle cell anemia; a 50 percent chance of inheriting the sickle cell trait (in this case, the baby will probably be healthy, but will be a carrier and have red blood cells containing some hemoglobin S); and a 25 percent chance of inheriting two copies of the normal hemoglobin.

According to the Sickle Cell Association of America, the disease began in at least four places in equatorial Africa, India, and Saudi Arabia. The disease then spread as people moved to other parts of the world. Today, both the sickle cell trait and

CGATTCTGAACATGATACGTACTGGTCCACTAGAACTGAACTCCAGAGGTACTAGA

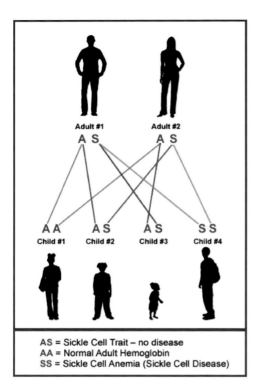

AS = Sickle Cell Trait – no disease
AA = Normal Adult Hemoglobin
SS = Sickle Cell Anemia (Sickle Cell Disease)

This chart shows the inheritance of sickle cell anemia with a "carrier" father and a "carrier" mother. A father and a mother who each have the gene for sickle cell anemia can pass the gene to their children. Every child has a 25 percent chance of having sickle cell anemia, a 25 percent chance of being healthy, and a 50 percent chance of being a carrier.

the disease exist mainly in people of African, Indian, and Hispanic descent and also in people from parts of Italy, the Middle East, and India.

Currently, sickle cell anemia is most common in West and Central Africa. According to the Sickle Cell Association of America, 1 to 2 percent of all babies born there have the disease, and as many as 25 percent of the people have sickle cell trait, which means that they are carriers.

Controlling Sickle Cell Anemia

People who have sickle cell anemia or trait can talk to a genetic counselor about the risks of having a child with the disease. A genetic counselor is an expert in genetic diseases.

TYPES OF SICKLE CELL DISEASE

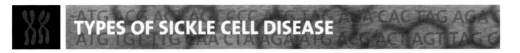

There are three main types of sickle cell disease. All types are caused by a genetic change in the beta globin part of hemoglobin. This genetic change causes sickle hemoglobin, or hemoglobin S, to form. Typically, a person receives two copies of the hemoglobin A gene. One copy comes from each parent. A person with sickle cell disease does not have copies of the hemoglobin A gene. People with the most common form of sickle cell disease have two copies of the hemoglobin S gene. Other people with the disease have one hemoglobin S and one other mutated hemoglobin gene. Many different types of hemoglobin disorders can occur less commonly with a copy of hemoglobin S. The three major types of sickle cell disease are the following:

- ◀ Sickle cell anemia, or hemoglobin SS disease, is the most common type of the disease. A person has two copies of the hemoglobin S gene.
- ◀ Hemoglobin SC disease is a rare type of sickle cell disease. A person has one copy of the hemoglobin S gene and one copy of the hemoglobin C gene. It is also called sickle cell C disease. The symptoms are milder than those of sickle cell anemia.
- ◀ Less commonly, a person can have one hemoglobin S gene and another mutant hemoglobin gene that causes thalassemia, another blood problem. This disease is also called sickle cell beta-thalassemia disease. Like hemoglobin SC disease, the symptoms are mild.

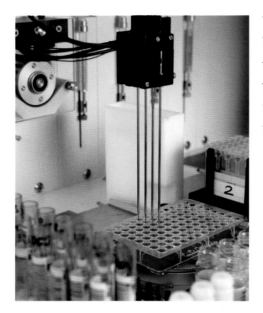

To test for sickle cell anemia, a blood sample is drawn from the arm. A machine similar to this one performs the test. The result will be either positive or negative for hemoglobin S.

If people do not know whether they have sickle cell anemia or trait, their blood can be tested for hemoglobin S. If negative, a person does not have the sickle cell gene. If positive, other blood tests can determine if a person has one or two sickle cell genes.

As of 2007, newborns in all fifty states, the District of Columbia, and the U.S. Virgin Islands are routinely tested for sickle cell anemia. A blood sample is collected from the baby's finger or heel and tested. A baby with one gene has a tiny percentage of hemoglobin S. A baby with two genes has a much larger percentage of hemoglobin S. A low red blood cell count means that the baby has anemia.

To test for hemoglobin S in an unborn baby, doctors sample the amniotic fluid. This fluid surrounds the baby in the mother's womb. A test can show whether or not the unborn baby is a carrier or has sickle cell anemia.

The next chapter describes the main symptoms of the disease and what it is like to live with sickle cell anemia. It also discusses current treatments, including the benefits and risks.

3

The main symptoms of sickle cell anemia are pain, anemia, and infection. Constant pain is the most common symptom of the disease. It can occur in any part of the body, but it most commonly occurs in the back, stomach, and joints. The pain can be mild to severe. A pain crisis, or an episode of severe pain, can last a few hours to a few weeks or more. Some people have a few pain crises during their life. Others have more than a dozen every year. A pain crisis can occur any time the sickled red blood cells block small blood vessels.

Sickle cells die much faster than normal red blood cells. The body cannot replace these cells quickly. As a result, people with the disease do not have enough red blood cells to carry oxygen

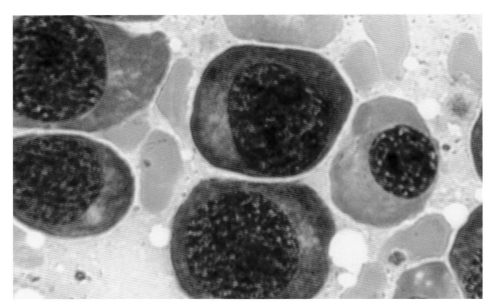

Red blood cells are made in the marrow inside the large bones of the body. This photo shows the bone marrow cells of a person who has anemia.

to tissues of the body. They then develop anemia. This causes them to feel very tired.

The spleen is an organ that fights infections. Because sickle cells damage the spleen, people with sickle cell anemia often get more infections than healthy people. They are also more likely to get serious infections such as pneumonia, lung disease, or bloodstream infections.

Other Serious Problems

Sickle cell anemia can damage all major organs and other body parts. This includes the kidneys, gallbladder, liver, eyes,

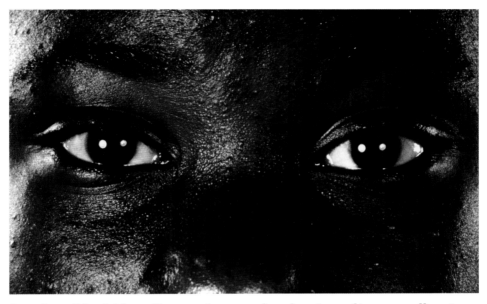

People with sickle cell anemia may develop jaundice, or yellowing of the skin and eyes. Jaundice results from the high rate of breakdown of red blood cells.

bones, and joints. Damage occurs from low oxygen or poor flow of the blood. Many problems can develop. For example, the lungs may not function well, so breathing becomes difficult. Damaged kidneys allow too much water from body cells to go into urine. Without enough water, body cells do not function properly. Because sickled red blood cells die too quickly, a lot of hemoglobin builds up, which can then form gallstones. Gallstones are painful, solid masses that form in the gallbladder or bile ducts. People with sickle cell anemia may develop jaundice, or yellowing of the skin and eyes, due to the accumulation of hemoglobin gallstones.

Red blood cells provide the body with oxygen and nutrients that it needs to grow. Having too few healthy red blood cells slows growth in children and in teens. People with the disease may develop vision problems. The tiny blood vessels to the eyes sometimes have too many sickle cells. This damages the retina, where light rays are focused. Consequently, people with sickle cell anemia may even become blind.

A stroke can happen if sickle cells block the flow of blood to the brain. During a stroke, a person may have seizures or difficulty speaking. That person may feel weak or numb in the arms and legs. He or she may lose consciousness. A stroke can result in death.

Another serious problem is acute chest syndrome. This condition happens when sickle cells are trapped in the lungs, or the person has a lung infection (pneumonia). Symptoms include chest pain, fever, and difficulty breathing. If the syndrome reoccurs, the lungs can become permanently damaged.

Sickle cell anemia can cause ulcers, or open sores, on the legs. This particular problem happens when sickle cells block blood vessels in the skin.

Being Careful

From an early age, people with sickle cell anemia must take special measures to manage their symptoms. They drink lots of water and reduce their exposure to the sun. These actions prevent dehydration and make it less likely for sickling to occur. Regular vaccinations, such as an annual flu shot and pneumonia shot, help to prevent these people from getting infections.

Many people take extra folic acid every day. The body uses this B vitamin to make new red blood cells. People with sickle cell anemia need to eat well-balanced meals. Healthy food gives the body nutrients to produce red blood cells.

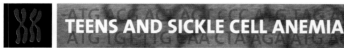

TEENS AND SICKLE CELL ANEMIA

Teens with sickle cell anemia have stresses including school, peer pressure, career goal decisions, and dealing with symptoms of this disease. Some may have body image problems. They often have delayed growth and puberty. They may not grow tall and may not develop much muscle. Coping with constant pain is tiring. Some teens fear opioid (narcotic) pain medicines because these medicines can be addicting. Living with sickle cell anemia is challenging because severe pain or other complications can start at any time. For support, teens can participate in teen support groups and/or have individual and family counseling.

Avoiding very cold or very hot temperatures is important. Extreme temperatures can cause sickle cells to form. Too much stress can cause tissues to lose oxygen and cause a pain crisis. Regular exercise can help to relieve stress. Too much exercise may be harmful because tissues may not get enough oxygen. Or, the person may overheat or become very tired. Any of these conditions can cause a pain crisis.

Treating Sickle Cell Anemia

Currently, there is no easy cure for sickle cell anemia. Although the transplantation of stem cells is curative, the procedure is not commonly performed because of the aftereffects and overall death rate. The goal of treatment is to manage symptoms and prevent complications from occurring. The type of treatment

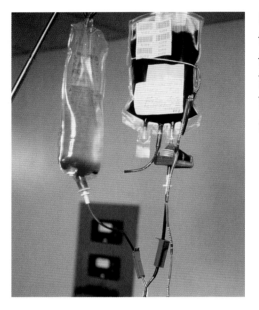

Blood transfusion is a treatment for sickle cell anemia. The blood transfusion bag that is hanging here is providing healthy red blood cells to someone with a severe case of the disease.

depends on the person and symptoms. For example, people need regular blood tests to check important labs such as hemoglobin counts. If these counts are low, the person may be treated for anemia. A person with an infection may take an antibiotic such as penicillin. Antibiotics treat infections caused by bacteria. Young children with sickle cell disease should also take preventative antibiotics, since their immune systems are not in the best possible condition.

People can take over-the-counter medicines for pain relief. For severe pain, they may need prescription pain medicine such as opioids (narcotics). During a pain crisis, a person may need to stay in a hospital and get pain-relieving medicines injected in the veins.

In 1995, Dr. Samuel Charache reported that the drug hydroxyurea, originally used to treat some types of cancer, could also be used to prevent some problems of sickle cell anemia. Three years later, the U.S. Food and Drug Administration (FDA) approved hydroxyurea as the first drug to prevent pain crises.

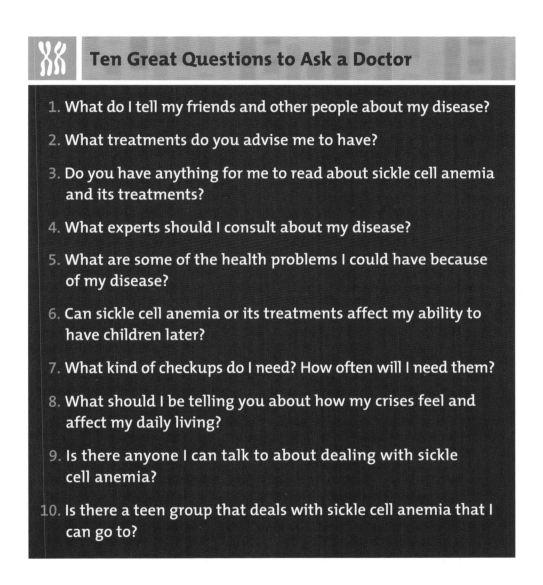

Ten Great Questions to Ask a Doctor

1. What do I tell my friends and other people about my disease?

2. What treatments do you advise me to have?

3. Do you have anything for me to read about sickle cell anemia and its treatments?

4. What experts should I consult about my disease?

5. What are some of the health problems I could have because of my disease?

6. Can sickle cell anemia or its treatments affect my ability to have children later?

7. What kind of checkups do I need? How often will I need them?

8. What should I be telling you about how my crises feel and affect my daily living?

9. Is there anyone I can talk to about dealing with sickle cell anemia?

10. Is there a teen group that deals with sickle cell anemia that I can go to?

Hydroxyurea acts by increasing the amount of fetal hemoglobin in red blood cells, which stops cells from sickling and blocking blood vessels. Generally, only unborn and newborn babies make fetal hemoglobin. Most fetal hemoglobin disappears by the age of six months.

CGATTCTGAACATGATACGTACTGGTCCACTAGAACTGAACTCGAGAGGTACTAGA

Today, some children and adults with sickle cell disease take hydroxyurea every day to reduce the number of pain crises, acute chest syndrome, and trips to the hospital for pain crises. However, taking hydroxyurea has risks. Over time, the drug may cause leukemia, a cancer of the white blood cells.

Pain crises require strong medicines for pain. People may need to stay in a hospital for treatment, and they often need intravenous fluids. They may also need extra oxygen, which goes to the blood and helps with breathing.

Blood Transfusions and Bone Marrow Transplants

People with severe sickle cell disease may sometimes need blood transfusions of non-sickled blood. This process gives healthy red blood cells to patients who are very prone to sickling and thus decreases the proportion of sickle cells in their bloodstreams. Sometimes, some of the blood from a person with sickle cell anemia is taken out before transfusing non-sickle cell blood. In a transfusion, normal red blood cells are removed from a donor, or volunteer. These cells then flow down a tube into the person with sickle cell anemia through a needle placed in a vein. The blood transfusion increases the number of normal red blood cells. After the transfusion, the person usually feels more energetic. The transfusion also decreases the chance of having a pain crisis.

Currently, blood transfusion is used for people with sickle cell anemia and other serious health problems. Blood transfusions can have potentially serious risks, though. People can get infections (most commonly, viruses) from the donated cells, although careful screening in the United States makes this problem much less likely. Other risks are the chance of developing a reaction to the cells of someone else or having the

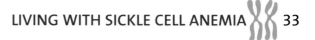

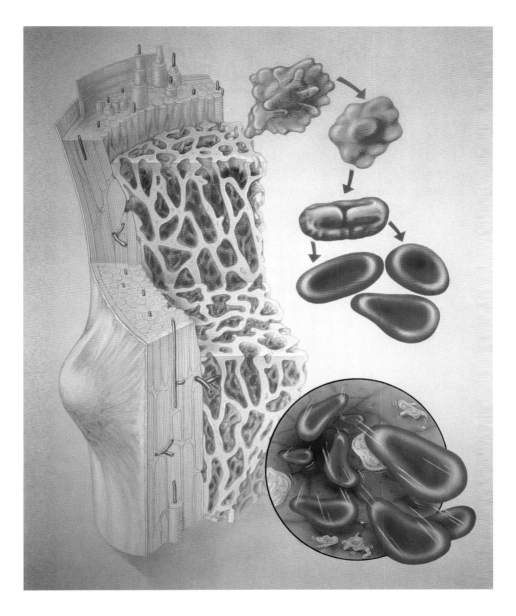

This illustration shows the bone marrow inside a bone and red blood cells. Red blood cells are made in the bone marrow of large bones. Bone marrow transplantation has saved some lives, but it is a high-risk treatment.

blood cells of the donor destroy the blood cells of the person with sickle cell anemia. Body tissues can also be injured from getting too much iron from normal cells if a person requires many blood transfusions. Too much iron can damage the heart, liver, and other organs. People who need regular transfusions often have to reduce their iron levels with medications. In 2005, the FDA approved deferasirox as the first medicine to reduce high iron levels in young children, although this medicine has been used in teens and adults for a while.

Bone marrow transplantation may be an option for people with severe sickle cell disease. In 1984, a child with sickle cell anemia and leukemia received a bone marrow transplant to treat the leukemia. The transplant helped the child's leukemia and sickle cell anemia. After that, a small number of people who had both sickle cell anemia and leukemia had successful bone marrow transplants. Doctors now treat only very serious cases of sickle cell anemia with bone marrow transplants.

Red blood cells are made in the marrow of some bones. In a bone marrow transplant, a person's own bone marrow is first wiped out by medicines and/or radiation. The healthy bone marrow is removed from a donor, often a sibling who does not have sickle cell anemia. The healthy marrow is given through a tube into the veins of the person with sickle cell anemia, similar to the way a regular blood transfusion is administered. The healthy marrow then starts to produce normal blood cells.

Like blood transfusions, bone marrow transplants are very risky. Sometimes, the transplant does not work, or the person's body rejects the new marrow. The person with sickle cell anemia must take medicines to prevent rejection of the new marrow. In addition, some people do not have a perfectly matched donor for the transplant. Currently, bone marrow transplants are used for only a small group of people with severe cases of the disease. Researchers are studying ways to improve these and other treatments for sickle cell anemia.

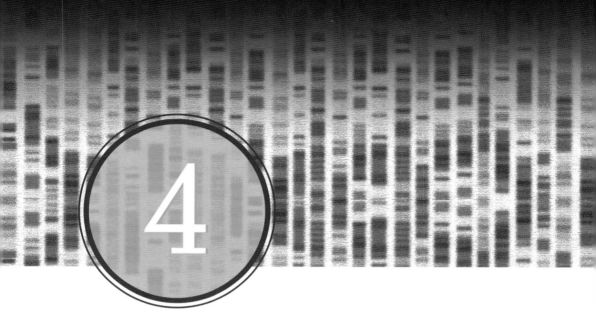

4

Modern research in sickle cell anemia is focusing on possible new ways of treating the disease. Some researchers are looking into helping the body make different hemoglobin. Others are studying ways to reduce sickling and increase the flow of blood. Researchers hope to find better ways for people to lead healthier lives.

Making More Fetal Hemoglobin

Fetal hemoglobin causes virtually no sickling. Unborn and newborn babies produce fetal hemoglobin. Babies start making hemoglobin S (a type of adult hemoglobin) between three and six months of age. Symptoms of sickle cell anemia then start to appear in people with sickle cell disease (two copies of hemoglobin S). Researchers are trying to find ways for people with sickle cell anemia to make more fetal hemoglobin to prevent the problems of having a lot of hemoglobin S.

Hydroxyurea is one medicine that has proven helpful for adults with the disease. The drug causes the body to make more fetal hemoglobin, which reduces pain and other complications. People then have less severe symptoms. Researchers are now studying the long-term safety of hydroxyurea in children and teens with sickle cell anemia. They want to determine how the drug affects their growth and development and whether children and teens can safely take the drug for many years.

Butyrate, or butyric acid, is a substance that can taste sweet and smell fruity. Food makers often add it to some foods as a flavoring agent. Scientists are studying the effects of butyrate in people with sickle cell anemia. They have found that it causes the body to make more fetal hemoglobin.

LIVING LONGER

Until recently, children with sickle cell anemia usually died young. According to the National Institutes of Health, about 50 percent of people with the disease now live past fifty years old. This is due to advances in treatment and management of the disease. Good pain management and treatment prevents infections and helps young people to develop and grow. They can help prevent complications of the disease by going in for testing and regular checkups with health-care professionals.

Reducing Sickling

Some researchers are looking into treatments to reduce the amount of sickling in the blood. Scientists are studying arginine (an amino acid, or building block of proteins) and its effects on sickle cell anemia. Arginine is found in the proteins that we eat, and the body makes it as well. Proteins are necessary for the structure and function of cells. Some scientists think that extra arginine may increase the levels of nitric oxide in the body.

People with sickle cell anemia have low amounts of nitric oxide, which is a natural gas in the body. Nitric oxide makes blood vessels become larger and red blood cells less sticky.

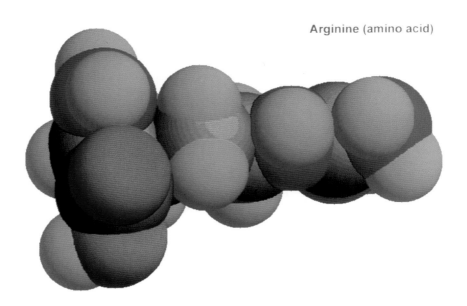

Arginine (amino acid)

Arginine is an amino acid that the body makes. It is found in many foods, such as dairy products, meats, poultry, seafood, and chocolate. It is also in wheat, oatmeal, nuts, seeds, and beans.

These conditions make red blood cells flow more easily. When red blood cells are broken down in the body, hemoglobin enters the bloodstream. Hemoglobin removes nitric oxide and can make blood vessels become smaller. Sickled and normal red blood cells move more slowly through smaller blood vessels.

Scientists are conducting arginine studies in adults and children. They want to see if extra arginine causes the body to make more nitric oxide. This could improve blood flow. Taking extra nitric oxide may mean that people will have fewer crises and less pain. They may not have to take as much pain medication.

Clotrimazole is an over-the-counter medicine used to treat fungal infections. Fungi are a group of organisms that include yeasts and molds. Clotrimazole also helps to prevent loss of

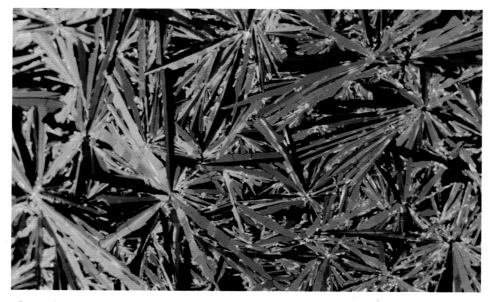

This photograph shows clotrimazole, an antifungal drug. It is used to treat skin infections caused by yeasts. Scientists are studying clotrimazole to determine whether this drug prevents sickle cells from forming.

water from red blood cells, which may help prevent sickling. Scientists are determining whether this drug reduces the number of sickle cells that form.

Scientists are testing vanillin to see if it will stop sickling in blood. Vanillin tastes like vanilla. Food makers often add it to cookies, cakes, and other foods. However, vanillin breaks down in the digestive tract before reaching the bloodstream. So, scientists have developed a special prodrug form of vanillin. A prodrug is a drug that turns into an active drug in the body. When tested in mice, prodrug vanillin helped red blood cells with hemoglobin S keep their normal shapes. Researchers have not yet studied the effects of vanillin in people.

Other Treatments

Children with sickle cell anemia often need more energy than children who do not have the disease. They may need to eat more food and eat more often. Children and teens with sickle cell anemia are often smaller and weigh less than those without the disease. They typically have less fat and muscle.

Researchers are studying whether children with sickle cell anemia can be helped by taking extra glutamine. The body makes glutamine, an amino acid that is a building block of protein. Scientists are studying whether children who take extra glutamine will have increased energy and growth.

Sickle cell anemia often causes damage to the blood vessels and nervous system. Sometimes, this condition results in strokes. People who have had strokes may have difficulty with movement or with processing information. Researchers are studying whether aspirin taken every day will lessen the chance of strokes and damage to the nervous system.

Another group of drugs that may help people with sickle cell anemia are statins. Some people take statins to lower their

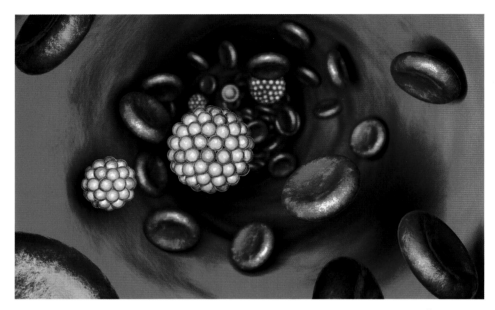

A blood vessel with red blood cells and balls of cholesterol (in yellow) is seen in this illustration. A group of drugs called statins lower the amount of cholesterol. Scientists are determining whether statins can help treat people with sickle cell anemia.

cholesterol. Cholesterol is a substance found in some of the fats that we eat. It is also made by the body. The body needs cholesterol to form vitamin D, sex hormones, and bile acids. Bile acids help the body to digest fats. Cholesterol is also part of the membranes of cells in the body. Researchers are determining whether statins can help people with sickle cell anemia. The statins may prevent damage to blood vessels by keeping nitric oxide at high levels in the bloodstream.

All the approaches covered in this chapter are a step forward in treatment. However, scientists do not consider them a cure for sickle cell anemia. The next chapter looks at new technologies aimed at curing sickle cell anemia.

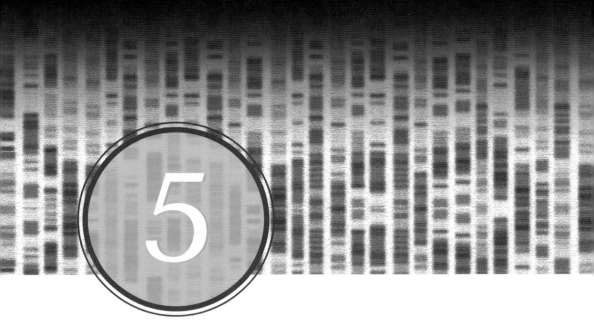

5

Genetic engineering, or altering the structure of genes, is key to the future treatment of sickle cell anemia. Molecular medicine scientists study the causes of diseases at the molecular level and then apply their knowledge to treat and prevent the diseases. Molecular medicine scientists change the structure and chemistry of molecules in the body. Because sickle cell anemia is a genetic disorder, it lends itself well to this kind of approach.

New Approaches for a Defective Gene

The ultimate goal is to find a cure for sickle cell anemia. One cure may be gene therapy.

CGATTCTGAACATGATACGTACTGGTCCACTAGAACTGAACTCGACAGGTACTAGA

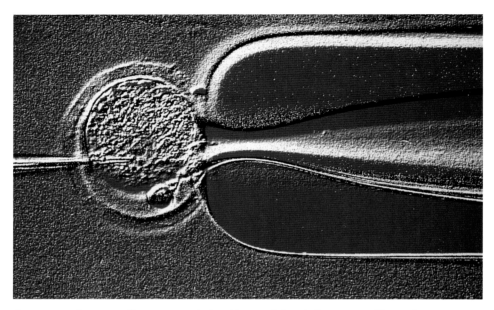

A researcher performs an injection of DNA into a cell to change its genetic material. The cell is kept stable by a suction tube *(right)* as the probe *(left)* injects the DNA.

By changing a gene or changing the expression of a gene, researchers may be able to treat, cure, or prevent a disease such as sickle cell anemia. "Expression" means to turn a gene on or off. Some researchers are studying how to replace a defective gene with a normal gene. Other researchers are studying how to turn off a defective gene or turn on another gene. The goal in all these approaches is the production of normal hemoglobin.

Sickle cell anemia is an excellent candidate for gene therapy. Unlike other genetic diseases, it is caused by one defective gene. Researchers have major challenges to overcome before they can use gene therapy as a cure. For example, they need to figure out how to insert a normal gene in a person with sickle cell anemia or how to change the effects of the sickle gene. This type of gene therapy is called somatic (relating to all of the cells in the body) gene therapy.

Somatic gene therapy could result in curing a person with sickle cell anemia. The cure would not affect the person's future children because the altered genes would not be passed to offspring. Offspring could pass the disease to their children. In germline gene therapy, scientists alter the genes in egg or sperm cells, and the person would pass the genetic changes to his or her offspring. Germline gene therapy could prevent a genetic disease, such as sickle cell anemia, from being inherited. However, not much research is being done in this area. Many people oppose germline gene therapy for ethical reasons. Also, the research work is very difficult.

EARLY STAGES OF GENE THERAPY

Gene therapy work is mainly experimental research conducted in laboratories. Although researchers have mapped the location of genes, they are just beginning to understand gene function. Currently, they know the function of only a few of the estimated 30,000 genes in a person. Gene therapy also has risks. Scientists often use viruses or other vectors (agents or carriers) to put a new gene into a body. These inserts could affect other cells and cause problems. A virus could be added to the wrong place in a DNA sequence and cause cancer or other health problems, even death. Because scientists do not yet know how genes are expressed, adding a new gene could cause too much protein to be made. As a consequence, too many red blood cells or a harmful protein could be produced.

Understanding Hemoglobin Genes

As a step toward understanding gene therapy for sickle cell anemia, researchers need to know how hemoglobin genes work. Recall that sickle cell anemia is caused by a mutation of the hemoglobin gene. Scientists at Virginia Commonwealth University are studying hemoglobin genes. Recently, they identified two proteins that regulate, or oversee, overlapping groups of genes during the development of red blood cells. Their findings may help researchers build gene therapies for people with sickle cell anemia.

Most people have two copies of the beta globin gene. This gene makes the beta globin in adult hemoglobin. People with sickle cell anemia have two sickle cell genes that make sickle cells. The two different proteins work together to regulate the globin genes responsible for the development of embryonic (very young) red blood cells. Embryonic red blood cells contain a lot of fetal hemoglobin that does not sickle.

The production of blood cells is a complex process. Globin genes regulate the process, and many molecules and proteins work together. Multiple globin genes are found on chromosome 11 in every person. These include gamma and beta globin genes. Beta globin is most expressed in adults. It combines with alpha globin (on chromosome 16) to make normal adult hemoglobin. In the development of the embryo, the embryonic globin gene is active, followed by activation of gamma globin genes in later pregnancy and in the newborn. The beta globin gene becomes active soon after a baby is born.

Gene Replacement Therapy

Understanding how genes are regulated is essential to gene therapy. Some scientists are studying whether a normal gene can be inserted into cells to correct the defective sickle cell gene. The hope is that the body would then produce normal adult hemoglobin.

Scientists can already make a normal beta globin gene in the laboratory. Replacing the defective gene with a normal gene seems like a good idea. However, scientists have to solve some difficult problems. One problem is how to have the body express high levels of the normal beta globin gene. Another is how to have the person continue to make normal beta globin. Yet another problem is that the remaining sickle beta globin gene would probably need to be turned off so that it does not produce sickle cell globins.

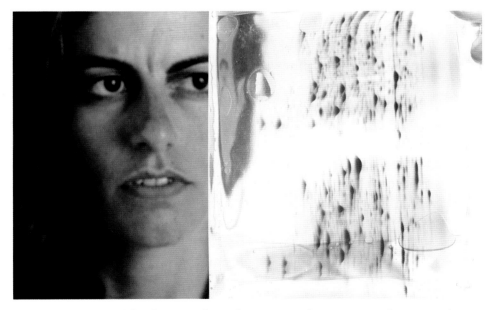

A researcher holds the results of a test to determine the proteins of an organism. Each dot is a different protein. Scientists are studying proteins to better understand genetic diseases such as sickle cell anemia.

Other scientists are investigating proteomics, the study of protein structure and activity. Proteomics is the focus of much research because it will help researchers understand the molecular basis of a genetic disease such as sickle cell anemia. This knowledge will lead to better treatments and possible cures.

Bone Marrow and Stem Cell Transplants

Currently, the only possible cure for sickle cell disease is a bone marrow or stem cell transplant. A stem cell is a very young, unspecialized cell in the body. It can grow into one of more than 200 specialized types of cells. Stem cells can make new stem cells or specialized cells. Bone marrow is rich in stem cells, which can become red blood cells.

In 2007, American researchers used a new process in stem cell transplants. They took skin cells from mice with sickle cell anemia. The cells were used to produce induced pluripotent stem (iPS) cells, which are similar to embryonic stem cells. The researchers inserted a healthy gene into the iPS cells and put them back into the mice. The mice began making healthy blood cells. These cells may someday provide a treatment or cure for people with sickle cell anemia.

Researchers have found that some people with sickle cell anemia can produce normal hemoglobin after having a bone marrow or stem cell transplant. Only a few people with severe sickle cell anemia have been treated with these transplants because they are very risky procedures. Researchers are working to reduce the risk by improving transplants.

Some researchers are studying a process called partial chimerism. During a bone marrow transplant, the bone marrow of the person with sickle cell anemia is usually

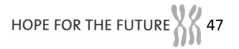

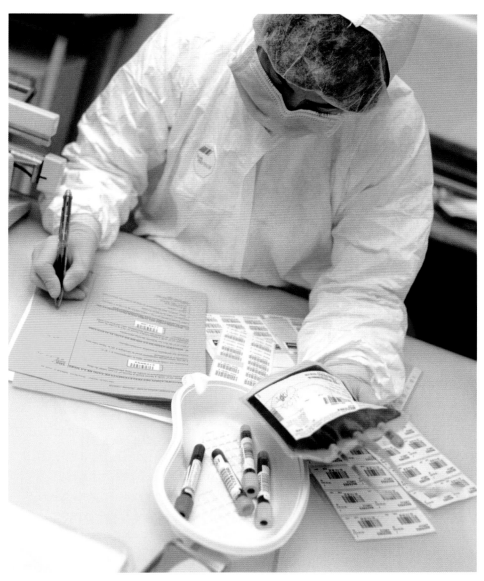

A researcher is preparing umbilical cord blood for transplant. Umbilical cord blood is rich in blood stem cells, which create red blood cells. Once stem cells are in bone marrow, they will create healthy blood cells.

destroyed completely, and a donor's bone marrow is given and takes over. In partial chimerism, the person's sickle cell bone marrow is not completely wiped out. A mix of the donor's non-sickle cell bone marrow and the patient's own sickle cell bone marrow exists after the transplant. Although some sickle blood cells remain, the person has few or no symptoms of sickle cell anemia. Fewer risks with partial chimerism exist than with full chimerism.

One area of sickle cell anemia research is using the blood from umbilical cords in stem cell transplants. The umbilical cord delivers food and oxygen to the fetus inside a mother's womb. The cord is rich in blood and stem cells. Researchers are finding that donors of cord blood do not need to match the person with sickle cell anemia as closely as bone marrow donors do. Cord blood could mean more potential donors for stem cell transplants. Unrelated people who donate cord blood may provide stem cells for people with sickle cell anemia. It may also reduce the chances of rejection and disease.

An Optimistic Future

Gene therapy is an ultimate cure for sickle cell anemia, but much work remains before it can be used. Meanwhile, advances in computer science are allowing researchers to model molecules and study how they behave. This approach allows scientists to screen for medicines that will most likely be effective in treating sickle cell anemia. With the sequencing of the human genome, researchers now are working to better understand the specific genes responsible for making proteins such as hemoglobin. This knowledge will allow them to perfect current technologies and develop new approaches. The future promises more effective and safer treatments, perhaps even a cure one day for sickle cell anemia.

Timeline

1846

The first modern description of sickle cell anemia is reported by R. Lebby, an American doctor.

1910

The first modern description of the symptoms of sickle cell anemia disease and sickled cells is made by James B. Herrick, another American doctor.

1917

Dr. Victor Emmel publishes a family history of sickle cell anemia.

1923

John Huck at Johns Hopkins University Medical School publishes the inheritance of sickle cell anemia through the generations of two families.

1927

Drs. E. Vernon Hahn and Elizabeth Gillespie at the University of Indiana show that low oxygen levels cause red blood cells to sickle.

1940

Dr. Irving Sherman at Johns Hopkins University Medical School reports that sickling of red blood cells without oxygen is caused by a change in the molecules of hemoglobin.

1948

Janet Watson, a physician in New York, finds that the blood of newborns does not sickle, which could be due to the presence of fetal hemoglobin in red blood cells.

Linus Pauling, an American chemist, shows that the hemoglobin of people with sickle cell anemia is different than the hemoglobin of people without the disease.

1956

Vernon Ingram and J. A. Hunt, scientists at Cavendish Laboratory at the University of Cambridge in London, map the amino acid sequence of sickle cell hemoglobin. Sickle cell anemia becomes the first genetic disorder in which the molecular basis is known.

1978

British scientist Richard Anthony Flavell maps the human genes that code for hemoglobin, demonstrating that sickle cell anemia is caused by a mutation in the DNA sequence of one gene.

1984

The first bone marrow transplant is used to treat a person with sickle cell anemia.

1995

Dr. Samuel Charache reports that the anticancer drug hydroxyurea reduces the pain of sickle cell anemia.

1998

The U.S. Food and Drug Administration (FDA) approves the use of hydroxyurea, which makes red blood cells less prone to sickling, for adults with sickle cell anemia.

2000s

Research begins into new ways of treating sickle cell anemia, including the interaction of proteins in regulating globin production, somatic gene replacement therapy, and more optimal stem cell transplants.

2006

A study sponsored by the FDA begins to determine if statins can help prevent injury to blood vessels.

2007

A study sponsored by the National Heart, Lung, and Blood Institute begins to collect, test, and store blood and DNA samples from children and adults with sickle cell anemia to study the role that genes play in the disease.

All states and the District of Columbia now routinely test newborns for sickle cell disease.

Researchers report that induced pluripotent stem (iPS) cells correct sickle cell anemia in mice.

Glossary

amino acid A molecule that makes up protein. There are twenty amino acids, and their sequence in a protein is determined by the genetic code in DNA.

anemia A low count of red blood cells. Anemia causes a person to feel tired and can occur because of various disorders or diseases.

chromosome A long thread of DNA encoding a series of genes and associated with proteins; chromosomes are found in the nuclei of cells.

deoxyribonucleic acid (DNA) The chemical compound that makes up chromosomes.

expression The functioning or activation of a gene.

gene A segment of chromosome that contains genetic information for a particular protein. A single gene or a combination of genes determines a trait, such as eye or hair color.

genome The entire collection of genes of an organism.

hemoglobin The protein in red blood cells that carries oxygen and is composed of four globin chains. There are different types of hemoglobin, including fetal hemoglobin and hemoglobin S.

hormone A chemical in the body that affects the way that other compounds or organs in the body behave.

induced pluripotent stem (iPS) cell An animal cell that is similar to an embryonic stem cell, but not exactly the same.

intravenous Performed or occurring within or entering by way of a vein.

jaundice The yellowing of the skin and eyes due to an accumulation of bilirubin, which is a product of broken-down hemoglobin.

meiosis The process that results in the formation of sperm and egg cells.

molecule A tiny particle consisting of two or more atoms held together by chemical bonds.

nucleotide The basic unit in DNA.

partial chimerism A mix of a donor's bone marrow and that of a person with a disease that results from a bone marrow or other stem cell transplant.

prodrug A drug that turns into an active drug in the body.

protein A type of substance found in all living things and that is composed of amino acids. Proteins are essential to the structure and function of cells.

stem cell An unspecialized cell in the body. A stem cell can grow into one of more than 200 specialized types of cells.

For More Information

American Sickle Cell Anemia Association
Cleveland Clinic/East Office Building (EEb18)
10300 Carnegie Avenue
Cleveland, OH 44106
(216) 229-8600
Web site: http://www.ascaa.org
Founded in 1971, the American Sickle Cell Association is the oldest sickle cell
research, education, and social services organization in the United States.

Anemia Institute National Office
151 Bloor Street West, Suite 600
Toronto, ON M5S 1S4
Canada
(416) 969-7431
(877) 992-6364
Web site: http://www.anemiainstitute.org
The Anemia Institute generates and shares knowledge about anemia,
especially among patients and health-care professionals dealing with
disease or treatment-related risks factors for anemia.

National Heart, Lung, and Blood Institute
National Institutes of Health
31 Center Drive MSC 2486

Building 31, Room 5A52
Bethesda, MD 20892
(301) 592-8573
Web site: http://www.nhlbi.nih.gov/index.htm
The National Heart, Lung, and Blood Institute provides leadership for a
national program in diseases of the heart, blood vessels, lung, and blood.
The institute conducts research and provides education.

National Organization for Rare Disorders
55 Kenosia Avenue
P.O. Box 1968
Danbury, CT 06813-1968
(800) 999-6673
Web site: http://www.rarediseases.org
The National Organization for Rare Disorders is a federation of voluntary
health organizations dedicated to helping people with rare diseases
and assisting the organizations that serve them. It is committed to the
identification, treatment, and cure of rare disorders through programs of
education, advocacy, research, and service.

Sickle Cell Association of Ontario
3199 Bathurst Street, Suite 202
Toronto, ON M6A 2B2
Canada
(416) 789-2855
Web site: http://www.sicklecellontario.com/frameset.html
The Sickle Cell Association of Ontario works to improve the health and
social well-being of individuals and families who are coping with sickle
cell disease.

Sickle Cell Disease Association of America, Inc.
231 East Baltimore Street, Suite 800
Baltimore, MD 21202
(800) 421-8453
Web site: http://www.sicklecelldisease.org

The Sickle Cell Disease Association of America promotes finding a universal cure for sickle cell anemia, while improving the quality of life for individuals and families who are dealing with the disease. This organization provides research, education, and services.

Sickle Cell Information Center
Grady Memorial Hospital
P.O. Box 109
80 Jesse Hill Jr. Drive SE
Atlanta, GA 30303
(404) 616-3572
Web site: http://www.scinfo.org
The Sickle Cell Information Center provides education, news, research, and sickle cell resources.

Web Sites

Due to the changing nature of Internet links, Rosen Publishing has developed an online list of Web sites related to the subject of this book. This site is updated regularly. Please use this link to access the list:

http://www.rosenlinks.com/gddd/scan

For Further Reading

Harris, Jacqueline L. *Sickle Cell Disease.* Breckenridge, CO: Twenty-First Century Books, 2001.

Huegel, Kelly. *Young People and Chronic Illness.* Minneapolis, MN: Free Spirit, 1998.

LeVert, Suzanne. *Teens Face to Face with Chronic Illness.* Englewood Cliffs, NJ: Silver Burdett Press, 1993.

Naff, Clay Farris, ed. *Gene Therapy.* Farmington Hills, MI: Greenhaven, 2005.

Panno, Joseph. *Gene Therapy: Treating Disease by Repairing Genes.* New York, NY: Facts On File, 2004.

Peak, Lizabeth. *Sickle Cell Disease.* San Diego, CA: Lucent Books, 2007.

Silverstein, Alvin, Virginia B. Silverstein, and Laura Silverstein Nunn. *The Sickle Cell Anemia Update.* Berkeley Heights, NJ: Enslow Publishers, 2006.

Bibliography

Achia-Abraham, Sathya. "Teamwork Between Two Key Proteins Necessary for Normal Development and Regulation of Red Blood Cells." Retrieved August 6, 2007 (http://www.news.vcu.edu/news.aspx?v=detail&nid=2162).

American Family Physician. "Sickle Cell Disease." Retrieved July 26, 2007 (http://www.aafp.org/afp/20000901/1027ph.html).

Anderson, Nina. "Hydroxyurea Therapy: Improving the Lives of Patients with Sickle Cell Disease." *Pediatric Nursing*, Vol. 32, Issue 6, November/December 2006, pp. 541–543.

Ascenzi, John. "Vanilla May Have a Future in Sickle Cell Treatment." Children's Hospital of Philadelphia. September 21, 2004. Retrieved July 25, 2007 (http://www.medicalnewstoday.com/articles/13729.php).

Basu, Priyadarshi, Pamela E. Morris, Jack L. Haar, Maqsood A. Wani, Jerry B. Lingrel, Karin M. L. Gaensler, and Joyce A. Lloyd. "KLF2 Is Essential for Primitive Erythropoiesis and Regulates the Human and Murine Embryonic ß-like Globin Genes in Vivo." *Blood*, Vol. 106, No. 7, October 1, 2005, pp. 2,566–2,571.

Bojanowski, Jennifer, and Rebecca J. Frey. "Sickle Cell Disease." *The Gale Encyclopedia of Medicine*. Record No.: DU2601001701. Health Wellness Resource Center.

Farmington Hills, MI: Thomson Gale, 2006. Retrieved August 2, 2007 (http:// infotrac.galegroup.com).

Bridges, Kenneth R. "A Brief History of Sickle Cell Anemia." Information Center for Sickle Cell Anemia and Thalassemia Disorders. Retrieved July 26, 2007 (http://sickle.bwh. harvard.edu/scd_history.html).

Bridges, Kenneth R. "Management of Patients with Sickle Cell Disease." Information Center for Sickle Cell Anemia and Thalassemia Disorders. Retrieved July 31, 2007 (http:// sickle.bwh.harvard.edu/scdmanage.html#gene).

Dolan DNA Learning Center. "Sickle Cell Disease: Your Genes, Your Health." Cold Spring Harbor Laboratory. Retrieved July 26, 2007 (http://yourgenesyourhealth.org/sickle/ whatisit.htm).

Dunayer, Eric. "Increased Understanding of Sickle-Cell Anemia: A Result of Clinical and In Vitro Research." *Perspectives on Medical Research*, Vol. 4, 1993. Retrieved July 24, 2007 (http://www.curedisease.com/Perspectives/vol_4_1993/ sickle_cell.htm).

Forbes.com. "New Kind of Stem Cells Reverse Sickle Cell Anemia." December 6, 2007. Retrieved December 6, 2007 (http://www.forbes.com/forbeslife/health/feeds/hscout/ 2007/12/06/hscout610648.html).

Frenette, Paul S., and George F. Atweh. "Sickle Cell Disease: Old Discoveries, New Concepts, and Future Promise." *The Journal of Clinical Investigation*, Vol. 117, No. 117, April 2, 2007, pp. 850–858.

Herrick, J. B. "Peculiar Elongated and Sickle-Shaped Red Blood Corpuscles in a Case of Severe Anemia." Archives of Internal Medicine, Vol. 6, 1910, pp. 517–521.

Hwang, Mi Young. "Facts About Sickle Cell Anemia." *Journal of the American Medical Association*, Vol. 281, 1999, p. 1,768.

Innvista.com. "Sickle Cell History." Retrieved July 26, 2007 (http:// www.innvista.com/health/ailments/anemias/sickhist.htm).

James, Thomas N. "Homage to James B. Herrick: A Contemporary Look at Myocardial Infarction and at Sickle-Cell Heart Disease." *Circulation*, Vol. 101, 2000, p. 1,874.

Kaye, Celia I., and Committee on Genetics. Newborn Screening Fact Sheets. *Pediatrics*, Vol. 118, No. 3, September 2006, pp. 1,304–1,312.

MedlinePlus Medical Encyclopedia. "Sickle Cell Anemia." Retrieved July 27, 2007 (http://www.nlm.nih.gov/medlineplus/ency/article/000527.htm#Causes,%20 incidence,%20and%20risk%20factors).

National Heart, Lung, and Blood Institute. "What Is Sickle Cell Anemia?" Retrieved July 27, 2007 (http://www.nhlbi. nih.gov/health/dci/Diseases/Sca/SCA_WhatIs.html).

Natural Sciences Learning Center, Washington University. "Discovery and Biological Basis of Sickle Cell Anemia." Retrieved July 28, 2007 (http://www.nslc.wustl.edu/ sicklecell/part1/background.html).

PBS.org. "Red Gold: The Epic Story of Blood." Retrieved July 28, 2007 (http://www.pbs.org/wnet/redgold/history/timeline1.html).

Pollack, Andrew. "Death in Gene Therapy Treatment Is Still Unexplained." *New York Times.* Retrieved September 21, 2007 (http://www.nytimes.com/2007/09/18/health/ 18gene.html?ref=us).

"Practical Tips for Preventing a Sickle Cell Crisis." *American Family Physician*, Vol. 62, No. 5, 2000, p. 1,363.

Quinn, C. T., Z. R. Rogers, and G. R. Buchanan. "Survival of Children with Sickle Cell Disease." *Blood*, Vol. 103, No. 11, 2004, pp. 4,023–4,027.

Showen, Nancy. "Sickle Cell Anemia." Retrieved July 25, 2007 (http://www.babycenter.com/0_sickle-cell-anemia_ 1422335.bc?Ad=com.bc.common.AdInfo%40230afbd0.

Sickle Cell Disease Association of America. "Who Is Affected?" Retrieved July 25, 2007 (http://www.sicklecelldisease.org/ about_scd/affected1.phtml).

U.S. Department of Energy Office of Science. "The Science Behind the Human Genome Project." Retrieved July 25, 2007 (http://www.ornl.gov/sci/techresources/Human_ Genome/project/info.shtml).

Washington State Department of Health. "Sickle Cell Anemia: A Parent's Guide for the School Age Child." Retrieved July 25, 2007 (http://www.doh.wa.gov/EHSPHL/PHL/ Newborn/scpg.ht).

Wethers, Doris L. "Sickle Cell Disease in Childhood: Part I. Laboratory Diagnosis, Pathophysiology and Health Maintenance." *American Family Physician*, Vol. 62, No. 5, 2000, pp. 1,013–1,020, 1,027–1,028.

Wethers, Doris L. "Sickle Cell Disease in Childhood: Part II. Diagnosis and Treatment of Major Complications and Recent Advances in Treatment." *American Family Physician*, Vol. 62, No. 6, 2000, pp. 1,309–1,314.

Wexler, Barbara, ed. "Genetic Disorders." *Genetics and Genetic Engineering.* Document No.: EJ3011370105. Opposing Viewpoints Resource Center. Farmington Hills, MI: Thomson Gale, 2006. Retrieved August 2, 2007 (http://infotrac.galegroup.com).

Index

A

acute chest syndrome, 28, 32
amino acids, 18, 20, 21, 37, 39
arginine, 37–38

B

blood transfusions, 32–34
bone marrow transplants, 34, 46
butyrate (butyric acid), 36

C

Charache, Dr. Samuel, 30
cholesterol, 40
chromosomes, defined, 16
clotrimazole, 38–39

D

deferasirox, 34
deoxyribonucleic acid (DNA),
    16–18, 19, 21, 43

E

Emmel, Dr. Victor, 10

F

Flavell, Richard Anthony, 21
Food and Drug Administration
    (FDA), 30, 34

G

gallstones, 27
gene therapy, 41–46, 48
genetics, science of, 16–20
genomes, 20, 48
Gilbert, Walter, 19
Gillespie, Dr. Elizabeth, 11
glutamine, 39

H

Hahn, Dr. E. Vernon, 11
hemoglobin
    defined, 13
    fetal, 31, 35, 44
    sickle (S), 15, 18, 21, 23, 24,
        35–36, 39
Herrick, Dr. James B., 9–10
Huck, John, 11
Human Genome Project, 20

Hunt, J. A., 18
hydroxyurea, 31–32, 36

I

induced pluripotent stem (iPS)
    cells, 46
Ingram, Vernon, 18

J

jaundice, 27
John Hopkins University Medical
    Center, 11, 13

L

Lebby, R., 9
leukemia, 32, 34

M

malaria, 10
Maxam, Allan, 19
meiosis, 18

N

National Institutes of Health (NIH),
    6, 14, 36
nitric oxide, 37–38
nucleotides, 16, 19

P

partial chimerism, 46–48
Pauling, Dr. Linus, 13, 15–16, 50
penicillin, 30
pneumonia, 26, 28
prodrug, 39
proteomics, 46

S

Sanger, Fred, 19
Sherman, Dr. Irving, 13
sickle cell anemia
    African Americans and, 6, 9–11,
        13, 14
    cause of, 21
    curing, 41–46, 48
    definition of, 5, 7
    early research into, 9–13, 15–18
    in history, 7–13
    inheritance of, 10, 11, 16, 21
    managing, 14, 22, 28–29, 31, 36, 39
    modern research into, 35–40,
        41–48
    myths and facts about, 14
    questions to ask about, 31
    statistics on, 6, 21–22
    symptoms of, 5, 6, 9–10, 25–28, 35
    teens and, 29
    testing for, 24
    treating, 29–34, 36–40
    types of, 23
Sickle Cell Association of America,
    21–22
sickle cell trait, 12, 21
statins, 39–40
stem cell transplants, 46, 48

V

vanillin, 39
Venter, J. Craig, 20

W

Watson, Dr. Janet, 13, 50

About the Author

Judy Monroe Peterson has two master's degrees, including a master's in public health education, and is the author of numerous educational books for young people. She is a former health-care, technical, and academic librarian and college faculty member; a biologist and research scientist; and a curriculum editor with more than twenty-five years of experience. She has taught courses at 3M, the University of Minnesota, and Lake Superior College. Currently, she is a writer and editor of K–12 and post–high school curriculum materials on a variety of subjects, including biology, life science, health, and life skills.

Photo Credits

Cover (top) © SPL/Photo Researchers; cover (inset) © www.istockphoto/ Chronos Chamalidis; cover (background left to right), p. 1 CDC, © www. istockphoto.com/Sebastian Kaulitzki; p. 5 © Educational Images/Custom Medical Stock Photo; p. 8 Courtesy of the Chicago Literary Club; p. 11 Indiana University School of Medicine Ruth Lilly Medical Library Special Collections; p. 12 © Kenneth Ewald/BioGrafx/Photo Researchers; p. 16 © Time-Life Pictures/Getty Images; p. 17 © Sam Ogden/Photo Researchers; p. 19 © Dr. G. Moscoso/Photo Researchers; p. 20 © Custom Medical Stock Photo; p. 22 Duke Children's Hospital; p. 24 © Tek Image/Photo Researchers; p. 26 © Michael Abbey/Photo Researchers; p. 27 © Welcome Trust/Custom Medical Stock Photo; p. 30 © SIU Biomed Comm/Custom Medical Stock Photo; p. 33 © Michel Gilles/Photo Researchers; p. 37 © Custom Medical Stock Photo; p. 38 © Michael W. Davidson/Photo Researchers; p. 40 © David Mack/Photo Researchers; p. 42 © Phanie/Photo Researchers; p. 45 © Mauro Fermariello/Photo Researchers; p. 47 © Burger/Photo Researchers.

Designer: Evelyn Horovicz; Editor: Kathy Kuhtz Campbell
Photo Researcher: Marty Levick

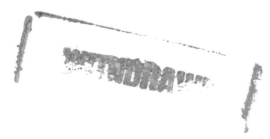